Food Myths

Joey Lott

CONTENTS

FOOD IS GOOD

I know what it is like to be terrified of food. In my case, I was nearly scared to death. I'm not exaggerating. Having heard and believed so many terrifying food myths, I had cut out one food after another, then entire categories of food, until I was down to skin and bones.

I'm not the only one, either. Since I finally came back to my senses and began to eat again, I have communicated with a *lot* of people who are similarly terrified of food. They've cut out all sugar, of course, because we all *know* how awful that stuff is. And they've cut out bread and all refined grains because we've heard over and over again how that stuff will kill us. And since grains contain all kinds of things like gluten and lectins and phytates, they've probably cut out all grains for good measure. They've also cut out butter, eggs, milk, and meat for all the reasons we've been told that these things are bad for us: cancer, heart disease, strokes, and so forth. And then they can't figure out why they feel so terrible – fatigued, irritable, bloated, nauseous, etc.

Of course, not everyone cuts out everything, but a lot of us have eliminated or restricted a lot of things, because we believe that we're doing the healthy thing. Maybe we've subscribed to veganism or to a low-carbohydrate diet. Maybe we've read *The China Study* or watched *Forks Over Knives*, and we've become convinced that animal fats and animal proteins are causing everything from cancer to diabetes. Maybe we've read one too many *Mark's Daily Apple* blog posts and decided that anything over 50 grams of carbohydrates a day will make us fat and then kill us.

My hope with this book is to take apart some of these myths. Whatever dietary camp you've subscribed to, I hope to at least plant sufficient doubt in your mind so as to free you from the dietary dogma that's been strangling you. My hope is that you'll be able to eat again.

The truth is that no one diet is the perfect diet for all people all the time.

1

Low-carbohydrate and ketogenic diets have value for some people some of the time. But for other people and at other times, they are the wrong diets. Likewise for vegan diets or low fat diets. Likewise for high protein diets and low protein diets. And yes, there may be appropriate times to manage sugar or salt intake, too. But for most of the people most of the time, these diets are unnecessarily restrictive, and as such, eventually they lead to poor health.

All the diets rely on myths to tell the story that convinces us to adhere to them. We become converts to the dietary religions, and so we believe in the myths. But that doesn't make them true. And when we dig in a bit, we find that none of them are actually *absolutely* true even on the rare occasion when there may be a kernel of truth to them.

Reality is that there are traditional diets all over the world that demonstrate that entire groups of people are able to enjoy good health with widely divergent macro and micronutrient ratios. Some traditions have relied extremely heavily on carbohydrates, including high glycemic carbohydrates, for their nutrition and energy. Others have relied heavily on animal fats and proteins. Some have gotten half of their energy from coconut oil. And still others have relied almost exclusively on dairy. And despite the sometimes radically different diets, these traditional diets supported groups of people who were free from cancer, heart disease, and diabetes.

The simple fact that very different diets that break all the "rules" of modern nutritional ideologies have worked well for people should in and of itself demonstrate that the myths we've believed aren't true. But in what follows, I offer you further evidence using modern research and studies that refute the myths. Hopefully, this will help you breathe more easily and enjoy your food.

Finally, it would seem that while food likely plays a role in our health, there may be other factors that are equally if not more important. Stress is a major one. So is how much we get outdoors in the sun. So is sleep.

Instead of being afraid of food, my hope is that this book may offer you reasons to love your food and enjoy your life. After all, it turns out that enjoying life and eating the food may be good for you!

So let's dig in. In the following sections, we'll look at one myth at a time. We'll start with sugar and carbohydrate myths, work our way through dairy myths, then meat myths, and finally some miscellaneous myths that are sometimes so crazy that they defy categorization.

SUGAR CAUSES CANCER

The "sugar causes cancer" myth is popular these days. Cancer is pretty scary to most people. Nobody really wants to get sick with cancer. And we want to have the security of knowing that we can protect ourselves from it.

Thus, the simple claim that sugar causes cancer appeals to us. Because we think, "Gee, I could give up sugar. It would be a noble sacrifice. And then I'd be safe."

Unfortunately, as we'll see, it's simply not true.

Sugar is the current dietary evil. It is enemy no. 1, regardless of which dietary camp one belongs to these days. So whenever something gets pinned on sugar, there aren't many who investigate it further and refute the unfounded claims. Nonetheless, there is no evidence that sugar causes cancer.

It is true that cancer cells use glucose (a sugar) to fuel themselves. Unfortunately, that is hardly enough to indict sugar for causing cancer, because *most* cells in the body prefer to use glucose as a fuel source. So claiming that sugar causes cancer is either naive or disingenuous. It would be more honest to state that sugar fuels cells. Period.

How does the body obtain glucose? Ideally from food. The body breaks down *any* digestible carbohydrate and converts it to the usable form of sugar – glucose. So whether you eat a banana, a potato, a piece of sprouted whole wheat bread, a piece of Wonder bread, a Frito, pancakes slathered in maple syrup, Lucky Charms, or a bowl full of white sugar, the carbohydrates get converted to glucose in order to be useable in the body. (Incidentally, I am *not* suggesting that all of those "foods" have equal nutritional value. I am merely pointing out that in terms of sugar, each is eventually converted to glucose.)

Advocates of the "sugar causes cancer" myth recommend eliminating all

3

sugar from the diet, in order to "starve" cancer. The problem with this is that in order to remove all sugar from the diet, one has to eliminate all digestible carbohydrates, including the much-beloved "healthy" carbohydrates such as carrots, beets, and beans. For low-carbohydrate or zero-carbohydrate advocates, this isn't a problem. They would love for everyone to stop eating carbohydrates, whether they come from Frosted Flakes or apples. The problem is that eliminating carbohydrates or even drastically reducing them not only starves cancer cells, it starves all cells, including healthy cells.

Once again, low-carb advocates suggest that this is not a problem – that it is, in fact, desirable. But it is not. Despite what the low carb advocates want us to believe--our bodies need glucose. Our bodies will even synthesize glucose if insufficient dietary carbohydrates are eaten. In other words, you absolutely cannot starve cancer cells of glucose while you remain alive since healthy cells and cancer cells alike use glucose.

Also, keep in mind that there are plenty of examples of groups of people eating high carbohydrate diets among which cancer is virtually unheard of. One such striking example is the traditional Kitavan people who have extremely low rates of cancer and yet eat 69 percent of their calories from carbohydrates (Lindeberg, Eliasson, Lindahl, & Ahrén, 1999). If eating carbohydrates (sugar) caused cancer, we would expect that groups of people who eat lots of carbohydrates would have higher rates of cancer. But they don't.

Timothy Moynihan of the Mayo Clinic speculates that the "sugar causes cancer" myth may be due to a misunderstanding of a common medical imaging test for cancer (Moynihan, n.d.). He points out that medical imaging uses radioactive glucose to look for tumors – not because cancer uses glucose preferentially, but because cancer cells use energy faster than healthy cells and thus concentrate *any* energy source.

Still, many who have an agenda grasp at anything that might support the view that sugar causes cancer. Thus, some claim that "because ketogenic diets cure cancer" we have proof positive that sugar causes cancer.

In the event that you aren't familiar with ketogenic diets, they are specially designed to deprive the body of carbohydrates and all but the minimum of protein so that the body is forced to use fat as the primary energy source. Some researchers are currently investigating whether ketogenic diets may be an adjunct to conventional cancer treatment (chemotherapy and radiation treatment) (Allen, et al., 2014).

That research suggests that depriving cancer cells of glucose creates additional oxidative stress in cancer cells *because using ketones as energy is not as efficient as using sugar.* Thus a ketogenic diet produces oxidative stress in all cells, but because cancer cells have faster metabolic rates it creates more oxidative stress more quickly in cancer cells.

There is nothing about that suggesting that sugar causes cancer. All it says is that sugar produces less oxidative stress than ketones, but because cancer cells have higher metabolic rates compared to healthy cells, using ketones in place of sugar is a "hack" that may increase the self-destruction rate of cancer cells faster than the self-destruction rate of healthy cells.

Furthermore, there is no evidence of which I am aware that demonstrates that ketogenic diets can cure cancer. I have seen at least one study that tested the impact of a ketogenic diet on advanced stage cancers (Schmidt, Pfetzer, Schwab, Strauss, & Kämmerer, 2011). Those who were able to successfully remain on the diet for the duration of the study showed mixed outcomes. Some minor positive outcomes were seen, but some problems were also encountered. Overall, the researchers concluded that ketogenic diets may be tolerable for some cancer patients, but nothing indicated that a ketogenic diet offers a miracle cure.

Also consider this: a Johns Hopkins study demonstrated that at least some cancer cells will adapt to use alternative fuel sources in the absence of glucose (Le, et al., 2013). Despite the apparent fact that cancer cells cannot use ketones as fuel, they are adapted to be able to use amino acids such as glutamine as an energy source. The implication is that in order to successfully "starve" cancer cells, one would have to not only eliminate all dietary carbohydrates, but also all dietary protein. Of course, the body would then begin to catabolize muscle and eventually even organs in order to meet its protein needs, which would inevitably feed cancer cells as well as other cells in the body. So this strategy of "starving" cancer cells is more likely to starve the person before it starves the cancer.

In conclusion, the claim that sugar causes cancer is completely unfounded. Sugar and carbohydrates in general appear to be an essential part of the human diet in most cases, and restricting them to "starve" cancer is misguided and potentially harmful.

SUGAR CAUSES INSULIN RESISTANCE AND DIABETES

Of late, the "sugar causes diabetes" myth has been circulating with virulence. In fact, the myth is now so loud and so overwhelming that just about everyone from the low-carb paleo diet adherent to the low-fat vegan to my middle American mother seem to conflate dietary sugar and insulin resistance, believing that the causation is so strong as to make the two essentially synonymous. The anti-sugar cult is shouting from the hilltops: "Sugar is making you fat, disrupting your endocrine system, and, in short, killing you."

But is it true? Is there actually proof that sugar causes insulin resistance and insulin resistant diabetes? I'll spare you the anticipatory anxiety and give you the answer up front. Simply put, no, there is no proof that sugar causes insulin resistance. Now let's dig in a little more deeply.

First and foremost, let's look at what insulin resistance actually is. As I've already suggested, insulin resistance is not as simple as "the effect of eating sugar," as we've been led to believe by the likes of Gary Taubes and Robert Lustig among the growing sugar haters. It turns out that insulin resistance simply means that the cells of the body are less receptive to the hormone insulin than ideal. Sometimes, this is what appears to be a natural and healthy adaptation given the circumstances (for example, ketogenic diets tend to produce insulin resistance, which may be advantageous given the sparsity of glucose in the ketogenic state). Other times, insulin resistance may be disadvantageous, as would appear to be in the case of type 2 diabetes when insulin resistance reaches a point at which insulin production cannot keep up and glucose begins to accumulate in the blood, causing many unpleasant symptoms and eventually death if left uncontrolled.

Before we get too much further, let's examine insulin itself. It is a hormone produced by the pancreas of a healthy human. Most of us are familiar (at least casually) with the idea that insulin is involved in blood sugar regulation – that insulin removes excess glucose (blood sugar) from the blood and it into cells for use as energy. But insulin also does a *lot* of other incredibly important things, including aiding the absorption of amino acids, preventing the breakdown of protein in the body (such as muscle), increasing blood flow, and increasing stomach acid production, to name a few. Because of this, it is important that the cells maintain an appropriate level of sensitivity to the hormone in order to maintain health. Still, for the purpose of this particular exploration, we'll be mostly concerned with the function of causing cells – particularly muscle and fat cells – to absorb glucose from the blood, which the cells can then use as energy.

Although we can view insulin resistance as a problem of insulin, there are other ways to look at it. When insulin resistance occurs, cells are less capable of taking in glucose from the blood. This may *not* be a problem of insulin or insulin sensitivity, per se. Instead, it may be an adaptation of the cell to prevent uptake of more energy than it can use. In this way of seeing things, we may instead interpret insulin resistance as a case of cellular respiration down-regulation. In other words, if there is a problem (which there may or may not be, depending on the circumstances), that problem may not be solved simply by forcing more glucose into cells. Instead, forcing more glucose into cells may cause cellular damage. And although tightly controlling dietary carbohydrates can *manage* the problem, it doesn't provide an answer. A better solution *may* be to improve cellular respiration so that cells can utilize glucose more efficiently. Keep this in mind as you read on, and it may shed some light on what follows.

What do the studies show to cause insulin resistance? Well, not much. There is little in the way of conclusive evidence of causes. In fact, perhaps the thing that is most strongly correlated with insulin resistance is excessive fat tissue around the midline, but researchers aren't even sure if *that* is a *cause* or a *symptom* of insulin resistance.

When we look at the effects of carbohydrates, the studies mostly show that more carbohydrates increase insulin sensitivity while fewer carbohydrates decreases sensitivity (Sargrad, Homko, Mozzoli, & Boden, 2005). This, of course, makes sense – the more carbohydrates one eats, the greater the efficiency with which the body would want to metabolize them.

So if carbohydrates (which includes both starch and sugars) can actually improve insulin sensitivity, then how does the link between a specific type of carbohydrate (sugar) and insulin resistance get made? Well, it turns out that the research *does* indicate that *excess* of one type of sugar – fructose – may cause insulin resistance in humans. This fact has caused many to jump on the anti-sugar bandwagon and start hating *all* sugar. But what do the studies *actually* say?

To begin with, let's look at the most damning of all, which is a study in which a group of healthy participants was fed 1,000 calories of pure fructose every day in addition to their normal diets (Beck-Nielsen, Pedersen, & Lindskov, 1980). The result? Insulin resistance in a very short timeframe (a week). So, apparently, eating 1,000 calories of pure, chemically-extracted fructose (which simply does not exist in any natural food) every day in addition to one's normal diet is probably a bad idea.

Okay, but in the real world, no one is going to do that. So let's look to see if there are any studies that show what high fructose intake does in slightly less obscene amounts. One such study showed that after four weeks, human participants eating 1.5 grams of fructose per kilogram of body weight (about 100 grams for a 150-pound person, which is approximately 400 calories worth of fructose) per day did not develop insulin resistance (Lê, et al., 2006). However, we don't know what might have happened if the study had gone on longer.

There was also a study done that showed that after six months, participants drinking one liter of sugar-sweetened cola (though the report says sucrose-sweetened, it is not clear if it is actually referring to sucrose or a sucrose-like product such as high fructose corn syrup, as is found in most colas) showed fat distribution in abnormal places, indicative of potential for future health problems (Maersk, et al., 2012).

So far, it seems that *really* high levels of pure, isolated fructose in addition to the normal diet can induce insulin resistance, yet lower amounts of fructose in the diet does not – at least not in a very short time. And we've seen that drinking a liter of cola every day for extended periods of time may not be a good idea, either. But how does one jump from these conclusions to another, more radical conclusion altogether – that sugar causes insulin resistance? Well, as it turns out, one has to simply make the leap without any credible support whatsoever, because there is no good evidence that sugar, on the whole, causes insulin resistance. There is only evidence that eating unnaturally high levels of free fructose can have that effect.

The trouble is that now the anti-sugar cult has grabbed the public and lured it into believing that *all* sugar is bad. I've seen claim after claim (all unsubstantiated) that fruit juice will cause insulin resistance. Many even go so far as to say to avoid whole fruits. And honey? That stuff is evil, we're told.

But here's the rub. It turns out that humans have been eating large amounts of fruit and honey for a long, long time without these foods causing insulin resistance and diabetes. In fact, there is good evidence that our earliest humanoid ancestors probably subsisted off of fruits, honey, nuts, seeds, insects, and scavenged foods. Many hunter-gatherer diets that have been cataloged rely heavily on fruit and honey for energy. And there's even a study that fed participants a diet of exclusively fruit and nuts for six months (minimum of 2,400 calories a day) (Meyer, van der Merwe, Du Plessis, de Bruin, & Meyer, 1971). The result? The participants experienced no health problems, and many reported greater feelings of stamina and overall health and well-being. Although the study wasn't explicitly concerned with insulin resistance, there were no indicators that the exceedingly high amount of fruit (and therefore relatively large amounts of fructose) caused any of the markers of insulin resistance. In fact, blood pressure (which is often high in insulin resistance) reduced among the participants.

So, despite the fact that many fruits are high in fructose (more than half of the sugar being fructose in some, such as apricots, oranges, peaches, and pineapples), it would seem that there may be some other factor in fruits that protects against whatever it is about pure fructose that can cause insulin resistance. Or maybe there's something about the process of isolating fructose that causes problems completely independent of fructose. Honey, also villainized by the anti-sugar cult for its high fructose content, is generally just fine. So there may be something in the natural sugar that is protective. And even sucrose, such as cane sugar, doesn't seem to be problematic in moderation, as shown by a study (Black, et al., 2006) that concluded: "a high-sucrose intake as part of an eucaloric, weight-maintaining diet had no detrimental effect on insulin sensitivity, glycemic profiles, or measures of vascular compliance in healthy non-diabetic subjects."

So if sugar isn't the cause of insulin resistance, then what is? Well, so far the research points to a few things as possible contributors – though as I have already stated, we can't point to any one thing and say, "That's what causes insulin resistance." Smoking is positively correlated with insulin resistance, as is a sedentary lifestyle. High stress (glucocorticoid production) is another factor. Inflammation may be a major player, and so anything that contributes to inflammation such as over-exercising, dieting, polyunsaturated omega-6 fatty acids, various forms of radiation, lack of sleep, and environmental pollutants may plays a role in contributing to insulin sensitivity.

In conclusion, it ain't the sugar, folks. But (in addition to all the other factors) it is possible that industrially-produced sugar products that are abnormally high in free fructose (such as most sodas) *may* be bad for health, particularly when consumed in large quantities on a regular basis. So stop villainizing real foods. They're not bad for you. Get outside. Smile. Get your bare feet on the ground, and play Frisbee or something. It'll do you a lot more good than avoiding fruit, honey, or even chocolate chip cookies.

SUGAR DEPLETES NUTRIENTS

One of the most popular anti-sugar myths, right behind the notion that eating sugar will necessarily lead to type 2 diabetes, is the idea that sugar depletes nutrient stores in the body, specifically B vitamins, magnesium, and calcium. Many like to use sensationalistic terms and suggest that sugar "robs" the body of nutrients. And some even make the claim that sugar will strip the bones of important minerals.

This myth is scary but unfounded. The truth is that I cannot find a single medical or scientific report that gives any credence to the claim. What seems to have happened is that some anti-sugar cultists have taken a basic metabolic fact and twisted it into an indictment of sugar without any merit. The factual statement would be simply that metabolism requires B vitamins, magnesium, and calcium. Whether one is eating a bowl of spinach, a bowl of Cheetos, a bowl of fried chicken, or a bowl of white sugar, the body is going to require B vitamins, magnesium, and calcium (and a whole bunch of other vitamins and minerals).

Of course, refined white sugar or refined white flour contains very little in the way of vitamins and minerals. In that sense, it is true that if one ate *nothing other than* white sugar or white flour, then there is a good chance that one would develop vitamin and mineral deficiencies. But then by the same token, we could select other foods that are deficient in one or more of the vitamins or minerals necessary for digestion, and make the same claims. In fact, by the very same argument, we could say that health-food darlings such as apples, spinach, and brown rice will all "rob" the body of minerals and vitamins.

Fortunately for most of us, we have more options available to us than white sugar and white flour. So we don't have to risk being nutrient deficient because we eat a mono diet. And the good news is that as soon as we eat a variety of foods, eating white sugar and white flour along with those other foods puts us at no greater risk of nutrient deficiencies than if we didn't eat white sugar or white flour, but instead only ever ate apples, spinach, and brown rice.

Specifically, let's look at some of the nutrients that are often cited as being of particular concern, i.e. the nutrients that the alarmists tell us that sugar will "rob" from our bodies. Of note are vitamin B1 (thiamin), vitamin B2 (riboflavin), vitamin B3 (niacin), vitamin B12, magnesium, and calcium.

As it turns out, the very best sources of B vitamins of all sorts, including B1, B2, B3, and B12 are animal foods such as fish, beef, lamb, pork, and eggs. Legumes, nuts, and seeds also have moderate amounts of many B vitamins, but *only* animal foods ever contain B12. Therefore, as it turns out, the only foods that don't "rob" your body of B vitamins are meats and eggs. Of course, I'm being facetious with this statement, but my point is that indicting sugar and flour because they aren't packed with high levels of B vitamins is a red herring. *Most* plant foods are lousy sources of B vitamins. Period.

What about minerals such as magnesium and calcium? Well, here the matter is also a bit tricky. Although many lists of good food sources of these minerals list various leafy green vegetables, nuts, seeds, beans, and whole grains, all of those foods contain substances (oxalates, phytates, and the like) that bind to the minerals, making them unavailable for humans. So the best reliable sources of these minerals are fairly few in number. For magnesium, decent sources include things like potato and banana, and for calcium, the best sources are dairy and bones. But it turns out that sugar cane molasses is one of the best sources of *both* minerals! So if you're concerned about deficiencies in either, then perhaps a spoonful of *sugar* molasses could be the best thing for you.

In conclusion, the anti-sugar contingent has twisted a fact in disingenuous ways to support the "sugar is evil" agenda. Eating white sugar or white flour does not "rob" the body of nutrients. All foods require nutrients to digest and convert into energy or muscle or fat or organs or anything else. White sugar and white flour provide large amounts of energy, which is necessary for the body to function, but do so without a great deal of vitamins or minerals. That is not inherently a problem, as long as they are eaten in the context of a diet that includes a variety of foods. Significantly, meat, eggs, and dairy all provide many of the essential nutrients necessary to digest food properly. That, combined with a spoonful of molasses, offers some nutritional insurance. Oh, and by the way, stress is the number one source of nutrient depletion. So relax. And enjoy some cake. It's good for you.

CARBOHYDRATES MAKE YOU FAT

Mark Sisson famously referred to 150+ grams of carbohydrates a day as producing "insidious weight gain," and Gary Taubes' best-selling book, *Good Calories, Bad Calories*, tells the reader over and over (and over and over) that carbohydrates make us fat. The believers of the Dr. Atkins dietary principles, the low-carbohydrate paleo philosophy, or any other low-carbohydrate or ketogenic dietary advice are all on board. But are they right? Will that baked potato, that piece of toast with a bit of jam, or the brownie really lead to "insidious weight gain," simply because of the carbohydrates?

Simply put, the idea that carbohydrates have some sort of superpower that inherently balloons up humans' midsections is absurd. There is no evidence to support this idea. The evidence is actually rather overwhelmingly *against* the theory that carbohydrates make people fat. In fact, research has shown that higher intakes of sugar are associated with *leanness* (Anderson, 1995).

One theory put forth as to why carbohydrates make people fat (which they don't) is the insulin theory. This theory states that insulin prevents people from burning fat. And since carbohydrates stimulate insulin increases in the blood the theory concludes that carbohydrates make people fat by preventing them from burning fat. This would be a good theory if it was tenable.

Unfortunately for proponents of the theory, it's not true, because in reality, things don't work like that. In reality, though one of the functions of insulin is to suppress fatty acid metabolism, it does so because it is prioritizing the metabolism of available glucose. Once glucose is no longer available, the body will resort to burning fatty acids. That's how it works. (That is, unless fatty acid metabolism is impaired.)

Let's say that you have just eaten a baked potato without any butter. I know it sounds pretty unappetizing, but you've done it for science. Once your body begins to absorb the carbohydrates, it will begin to produce insulin – a fair amount, as it turns out. Let's say that that potato has about 30 grams of carbohydrates that your body will break down into glucose. So your blood now has a bunch of glucose in it. The insulin will help move glucose into cells for use as fuel, and when it does so, it will be signaling the cells to stop burning fatty acids (if they have been) because glucose is available instead. Yay for insulin, because it has just done a great thing! It has fueled your cells with the energy from the food you just ate. Once the glucose from the food that was just eaten has been used, the body will then return to using stored fuel, whether that is glucose or fatty acids.

Next – again, in the name of science – let's say that you eat a spoonful of coconut oil. Being a fat, coconut oil doesn't trigger insulin secretion. Instead, as the fat is broken down and absorbed into the blood, the cells will use the fat as fuel. Once the fat is used up, the body will then return to using stored fuel.

Hopefully you can see that there is actually very little difference between carbohydrates and fat (the two primary fuel sources in the body) when it comes to the potential to increase fat stores. Basically, what is eaten gets used or stored. Then stored fuel is used. The insulin theory is bogus.

The other theory that is popular is the leptin resistance theory. This theory says that carbohydrates inhibit feelings of satiety and therefore lead to overeating, which causes obesity. It's a nice theory, but it's not supported by the evidence. While there is some evidence that *some* types of carbohydrates (think free fructose, for example) can have this effect, it doesn't extend to all carbohydrates. In fact, as we've already seen, carbohydrates trigger insulin secretion, and insulin triggers feelings of satiety. The studies bear this out in the real world. Carbohydrates (as in real food) don't make people eat past satiety, though specific types of industrial and refined carbohydrates may have such an effect.

Not only do studies show that carbohydrates don't make people fat, but real world examples of cultures that depend on large amounts of carbohydrates – sometimes as much as 80+ percent of calories coming from carbohydrates – demonstrate that they are generally lean, fit, and healthy. Consider the darlings of researchers, the Kitavans, who in the 1990s were shown to eat nearly 70 percent of their calories from carbohydrates (Lindeberg, Nilsson-Ehle, Terént, Vessby, & Scherstén, 1994). Obesity is non-existent in the population. Nor is insulin resistance found among the people, for that matter. And there are a great many other examples showing the same thing. Carbohydrates do not make people fat.

Interestingly, the same researchers who studied the Kitavans also showed that in though eating large amounts of carbohydrates, the Kitavan people had *lower* levels of insulin compared to European populations

(Lindeberg, Eliasson, Lindahl, & Ahrén, 1999). So once again, the claim that eating carbohydrates causes people to become fat through increased insulin levels is bogus.

What does make people fat? Honestly, we don't know. There are many theories, and none of them, as yet, can explain obesity in every case. Some factors that may contribute are yo-yo dieting, chronic stress, ionizing radiation, many pharmaceuticals, chronic insufficient sleep, and inflammation. And it does seem that there may be a link between certain types of industrial carbohydrates and obesity. Notably, free fructose as found in *very* high fructose corn syrup (added to sodas) may play a role, but that's a far cry from blaming carbohydrates as a whole. The evidence strongly suggests that sugars and starches found in real foods, even partially refined carbohydrates, are not inherently fattening.

HIGH GLYCEMIC INDEX FOODS CAUSE INSULIN RESISTANCE

Once the "carbohydrates are bad" myth wears thin, many people start to cling to various fantastical theories about why *some* carbohydrates are bad while *maybe* others are okay. Chief among these theories is the glycemic index theory.

The glycemic index is a concept that seeks to determine how quickly and to what extent a food raises blood glucose levels. Foods that produce a large and quick increase in blood glucose have a high index value, while foods that produce a small and slow increase in blood glucose have a low value.

The theory is that a diet with a large amount of high glycemic index foods significantly contributes to insulin resistance and diabetes. And like so many theories, it would be a good one if only it were true. But it is not. Let's look more closely.

As you may recall from earlier in this book, there is no causal link between carbohydrate consumption and insulin resistance except that, perhaps, insulin sensitivity can be reduced by consuming a very low carbohydrate diet. Glucose is *particularly* benign. And so a food like potato, whose carbohydrate content is primarily glucose, has not been shown to contribute to insulin resistance. Yet it turns out that in most glycemic index lists, potatoes have very high values. Therefore, according to the theory, potatoes should be causing insulin resistance on account of their high glycemic index value. But, as it turns out, they do not. And this is further reinforced by the fact that populations eating traditional diets that rely heavily on potatoes have low incidences of insulin resistance.

As you may also recall from earlier mention in this book, free fructose (as in refined, isolated fructose – something that doesn't occur in nature) *is* linked with insulin resistance, and extremely large amounts of free fructose fed to humans has been shown to produce insulin resistance in a very short time. But guess what? Fructose has a low glycemic index value. Not just low. *Very* low.

There are more problems with the glycemic index theory of insulin resistance. It turns out that the way in which individuals will react to foods varies greatly. In fact, how one person reacts to the same food will be different on different occasions, even under controlled circumstances (glycemic index values are measured after 15 hours of fasting). So the glycemic index values in a list are not necessarily good predictors of how *an individual* person will react *right now*.

What is more, the glycemic response to a food changes when combined with another food. For example, a potato may have a very high glycemic index by itself, but add some butter and it's a moderate glycemic index value. So even *if* high glycemic foods produced insulin resistance (and apparently they do not), you'd have to be eating lots of them *by themselves*. And very few people eat a bunch of plain, dry potatoes, rice, and corn flakes all day long.

Finally, the studies that look at the impacts of high glycemic foods on insulin sensitivity supply no evidence that there is any negative impact. Stephan Guyenet, who maintains a blog called Whole Health Source, compiled a list of long-term controlled trials that compare the impacts of low glycemic versus high glycemic foods. The studies showed essentially no significant differences in insulin or glucose control between low and high glycemic diets. The only study that showed any significant difference between the two groups was one that fed one group a high glycemic index, wheat-based diet and the other group a low glycemic index, rye-based diet. It seems unlikely that the difference noted in the groups was because of glycemic indices. Rather, it seems more likely that there may be some features specific to wheat and rye to which the differences can be attributed.

In conclusion, if the glycemic value of foods plays any roles in health, causing insulin resistance does not seem to be one of them.

WHITE FLOUR TURNS TO GLUE IN THE GUT

One of the myths that originally prompted me to write this book is the persistent myth that white flour turns into glue in the gut, binding, clogging, and coating the stomach and intestines. Those who make this claim often advocate for consuming whole grain flour or other whole grain foods instead of white flour foods. So is there any merit to the argument? And are the proposed remedies helpful alternatives?

The story that usually accompanies the myth makes it more believable. Most of us have created papier-mache at some point in our lives by using white wheat flour paste. Those who perpetuate the myth remind us of this paste and suggest that just as wheat flour paste can glue paper, it will glue our insides. At a very superficial level, this story makes sense, and therefore it is believable, so long as one does not scratch below the surface. However, it turns out that it simply is not true.

Gluten is a (now infamous) protein contained in wheat and some other grains, and it is gluten that is responsible for the glue-like properties of wheat flour paste. So it turns out that both white and whole grain wheat flour can be used equally for the purpose of creating paste for gluing paper, since both contain gluten. The gluten cross-links, forming a glue.

Gluten is actually a matrix of proteins, including glutenin and gliadin. Glutenin is a very long protein that is principally responsible for the glue-like nature of gluten. Gliadin, on the other hand, is compact and does little to form any glue-like substances. Let's next look at how the human body digests these substances.

Most of us these days have heard of gluten sensitivity or diseases such as Celiac disease, which involves problems with gluten. It turns out that for most people, the primary problem with gluten isn't with gluten as a whole, but specifically with gliadin, the compact protein that makes up part of the matrix. Gliadin can be difficult to digest because of its complexity and compact nature. And for *some* people (estimated to be somewhere in the range of 0.5 to 1 percent of the population) gliadin creates serious problems in the intestines. But remember, gliadin is not the protein that creates glue – that's glutenin. So what happens to glutenin in the human digestive system?

It turns out that enzymes secreted in the human digestive system – proteases that break down proteins – pull apart glutenin into amino acids. The intestines then absorb the amino acids.

So does wheat flour create glue in the guts? Nope. It does not, because glutenin, the protein responsible for the glue-like nature of wheat flour paste, gets completely digested.

By now, we've already seen that flour does not, in fact, create glue in the guts. But all the same, let's see if the suggestions made by those who promote that myth have any merit on their own. Namely, are whole grain flours or other whole grain foods better than white flour for preventing digestive problems?

A whole grain contains a bran layer, a germ, and an endosperm. When grain is refined, all that remains is the endosperm, containing mostly starch and some protein. Most people are completely capable of digesting the protein, starch, and any fats contained within the grain, so whether a grain is whole or refined, those parts will be broken down and absorbed. The endosperm will often contain some small amount of fiber that resists digestion by human digestive enzymes, but that fiber is typically fermentable, so it will be eaten by the bacteria in the large intestines. The only part of the grain that resists digestion both by enzymes and by bacteria is the insoluble fiber that makes up the bran.

If one is genuinely allergic or intolerant to a particular grain, then the presence or absence of bran will make no difference. For example, gluten, the protein in wheat and some other grains that can cause major health problems for a small percentage of the population, is contained in the endosperm. In other words, it remains once the bran has been milled away, but it also exists in whole wheat. So if someone has Celiac disease, both refined wheat and whole wheat are equally problematic. But for everybody else this is not a problem.

In conclusion, white flour does not turn into glue in the guts. And for the vast majority of people, white flour poses no special harm to the digestive system. Of course, some people have problems with gluten or allergies to various grains. In those cases, the problems are not mediated by the presence or absence of bran, so the recommendations made by those who perpetuate the glue myth are unfounded.

POTATOES HAVE NO NUTRITIONAL VALUE

The humble potato has been an important food staple in the diets of people worldwide. Originating in South America and domesticated perhaps 10,000 years ago, potatoes have been an essential part of the traditional diets of many native people of the Americas for a very long time. And since their introduction to Europe, many cultures, notably the Irish, heartily adopted potatoes as their own, immediately recognizing the tremendous importance of the food.

Yet despite the obvious value of potatoes, many have sought to denigrate them in recent years. As a result, it would seem that many people simply assume that white potatoes are nutritionally inferior to other foods. But as we'll see, that's simply untrue. In fact, ounce for ounce, potatoes pack in more vital nutrients than almost any other food! (King & Slavin, 2013)

These days it is common for "health-conscious" people to eschew "regular" potatoes in favor of what they imagine to be a healthier alternative: the sweet potato. Interestingly, despite the fact that there is essentially nothing any less "paleo" about potatoes versus sweet potatoes (or cabbage, for that matter), many paleo diet adherents forgo potatoes entirely. But is everyone right to hold potatoes in such poor esteem? Let's look.

Perhaps the most significant nutritional contribution of a potato is the starch content. A "medium" potato (about 150 grams) contains around 25 grams of starch. Although there is a strong anti-starch/anti-carbohydrate sentiment among many these days, the starch content of potatoes is probably a major reason for their tremendous importance among traditional cultures, because they recognized the importance of food energy. Potatoes provide a lot of energy, which is a very good thing for those who wish to remain alive.

But potatoes provide much more than starch. They also provide protein. That same medium potato packs in just over 4 grams of protein. And what makes potato protein especially important is its quality. Among plants, potato protein may be the very highest quality – so much so that it is conceivable to survive on potatoes alone. The same cannot be said of most any other plant proteins.

In the vitamin department, potatoes aren't too shabby. A medium potato offers up 50 percent of the U.S. daily recommended amount of vitamin C, and it yields 30 percent for vitamin B-6. Compare that to a sweet potato, and already the standard spud is looking mighty good. But there's more, because that same potato also yields a substantial serving of other B vitamins.

What about minerals? Again, the potato is nothing to laugh at. That medium potato has nearly 900 mg of potassium – more than any other vegetable on an ounce per ounce basis. That potato also contains a moderate dose of magnesium plus a fair amount of copper and manganese.

When Women Infants and Children (WIC) decided to remove potatoes from the approved foods, Chris Voigt, executive director of the Washington State Potato Commission, decided to eat nothing but potatoes for two months in order to demonstrate the nutritional value of potatoes. He managed to gain a lot of good publicity for potatoes as a result. In the 60 days, his fasting glucose level dropped 10 points and his cholesterol levels, triglyceride levels, and blood pressure all dramatically improved. He demonstrated what people have known for thousands of years: potatoes are nutritious, healthy food.

So next time someone denigrates the potato, you can smile inwardly, knowing that you're doing your body good by enjoying the nutritious tuber. And when you add some equally nutritious butter and salt to the equation, you've got something pretty darn delicious.

CASEIN IS BAD

Casein is a protein found in milk and many dairy products. It is the protein that curdles, forming cheese. And it has gotten a bad rap. Like gluten, a protein in wheat, casein *can* be problematic for *some* people. Some people speculate that casein sensitivities may be involved in creating problems for those with autism – something as yet unproven but at least plausible. Unfortunately, this speculation has been extended to the general population, and now a lot of people eliminate dairy because they are concerned about casein.

Is casein really so bad? In a word, no, it is not.

In 1991, a Norwegian doctor named Kalle Reichelt hypothesized that casein (and gluten) may play a role in autism. He claimed that those with autism have different patterns of peptides in their urine when compared to those without autism, and based on that, he speculated that casein (and gluten) may be incompletely digested in those with autism, and they may be wreaking havoc, specifically at opioid receptors in the body.

As a result, gluten-free, casein-free diets are now commonly employed in an effort to treat autism. However, these diets still are not validated by studies. Of course, there are some positive outcomes on these diets for some people, but whether or not that is because of some inherent problem with casein remains unclear. Furthermore, it is a mistake to generalize any such theory to the whole population.

The evidence is that, at least for the overwhelming majority of people, casein poses no problems. Not only that, but casein has some significant benefits. For one thing, casein is a high quality protein, and particularly when combined with whey in milk, the protein quality is exceptional. Casein is unique among proteins in that it is both high quality and it digests very slowly. This is beneficial because it keeps the levels of circulating amino acids high. The result is that casein has a uniquely anabolic quality. This is very important for those who are recovering from exercise, injury, or illness.

Finally, scientists have now identified two genetic variants among dairy cows: A1 and A2. There is now some belief that only A1 casein has the potential for producing problems. Meanwhile, A2 casein may not only not be problematic, but it may be downright healthy. In a review of the matter (Bell, Grochoski, & Clarke, 2006) the authors state: "Populations which consume milk containing high levels of ss-casein A2 variant have a lower incidence of cardiovascular disease and type 1 diabetes. Furthermore, consumption of milk with the A2 variant may be associated with less severe symptoms of autism and schizophrenia."

The implications of A1 versus A2 variants are still not clear, and it may be that the differences aren't significant at all for the general population. In fact, in the same review (Bell, Grochoski, & Clarke, 2006) the authors go on to state that while infants may absorb the theoretically problematic fraction of A1 milk, adults do not.

However, with all that said, if you are interested in seeking out milk from A2 cows, then you may want to find a small, local dairy farm with Jersey, Guernsey, or Brown Swiss cows, all of whom are predominantly A2.

DAIRY IS LIKE HEROIN

In recent years, some research has come out demonstrating that casein in cow's milk may sometimes break down into peptides called casomorphins. These peptides have opioid structures, leading to the popular (though as of yet unfounded) conclusion that dairy may act like opioids in the human body. Soon the headlines were flying with absurd claims that cheese is like heroin. Some even stupider claims suggest that cheese may be akin to crack cocaine – a comparison that misses the point entirely, since crack cocaine is not an opioid. And the vegan advocates didn't miss the opportunity to remind us, "See, we told you that milk is bad!"

But is it true? Is dairy really bad for us because of casomorphins? It would seem that by and large the answer is no. Let's look into this myth a little further.

As we saw in the previous section, milk contains a protein called casein. Under some circumstances, casein can break down into peptides called casomorphins, which have the structure of opioids. The casomorphin that has received the most attention and the one that is blamed (without any evidence to back up the claim) for everything from autism to cancer is beta-casomorphin-7 (BCM7), which can only be formed from milk from cows with the A1 genetic variant. So at this point, the *only* concern that has been raised is specific to BCM7.

Of interest is that with one exception, the published papers on the subject of BCM7 do not show harmful effects. In fact, they report immuno-modulatory effects. Not only that, but a series of studies (Zhang, Miao, Wang, & Zhang, 2013) show a whole host of protective benefits of BCM7 in diabetic rats. Of course, these are rat studies, and the results don't always translate well to humans.

The only study claiming that BCM7 is potentially harmful (Tailford,

Berry, Thomas, & Campbell, 2003) would be less misleading if the following phrase was added to the title: *in rabbits*. Perhaps the authors weren't aware of the fact that rabbits are herbivores, meaning that animal fats and proteins are unnatural for adult rabbits. And while no studies involving non-human animals will give an accurate picture of the effects on humans, rabbits are particularly different than humans, whereas rats have more similarities.

That casomorphin should be benign or potentially beneficial for the majority of humans is not surprising. Although the sensationalistic headlines liken casomorphin to heroin, creating a negative association for most people, the reality is that there are a *lot* of different naturally-occurring opioids that provide valuable benefits to human health.

For one thing, human breast milk contains the human version of BCM7, and there are various investigations into the potential benefits of BCM7 for human infants. Based on the current research, it is reasonable to believe that BCM7 may provide important immuno-modulating properties to the newborn infant with an immature immune system. So the idea that BCM7 is inherently bad turns out to be unfounded.

For another thing, the human body produces lots of opioids naturally. Perhaps the most famous type of endogenous opioid is the endorphin, but there are others, including enkephalins, dynorphins, and endomorphins. All of these substances produced naturally in the body provide important health benefits ranging from pain relief to appetite regulation to immune modulation to sleep and temperature regulation. So it is disingenuous to suggest that all opioids are necessarily bad for health.

Oh, and another thing, despite the emphasis on casomorphins, which are opioid agonists, dairy also contains opioid antagonists. That means that milk contains substances that naturally oppose the actions of BCM7. These substances are not well studied, so not a lot can be said about them, but it is reasonable to assume that there is some sort of balancing act that goes on.

Of course, it would be similarly disingenuous to suggest that casomorphins and specifically BCM7 are always perfectly benign. Some people may react badly to them. In particular, it seems that those with increased intestinal permeability may be at risk for negative effects. So some people may genuinely be better off, at least in the short term, without A1 dairy foods in their diets. And anyone concerned about any potential negative effects who still wants to include dairy in their diet may want to seek out A2 milk from traditional breeds of cows.

LACTOSE IS BAD

Lactose is a disaccharide (a sugar composed of two simpler sugars) found in milk that has gotten a bad rap. Anti-dairy folk like to point out that as much as two-thirds to three-quarters of the world's adult population don't produce much lactase, the enzyme that breaks down lactose. And they often go on to paint a scary story about the implications of lactose intolerance and the negative health consequences. As a result, some people avoid dairy altogether.

Lactose naturally occurs in all milk, including human breast milk. In fact, breast milk contains significantly higher quantities of lactose when compared to cow's milk. Infants naturally secrete an enzyme called lactase that breaks lactose apart into simpler sugars, glucose and galactose, both of which the body can absorb and use. So for anyone who produces lactase, lactose is perfectly easy to digest.

The (imagined) problem occurs when a person does not create lactase. In certain areas of the world (Europe, East Africa, and West and South Asia [the Middle East and Indian subcontinent]), humans evolved to continue to produce lactase into adulthood. These are regions in which humans have long relied upon milk as a significant part of their diet. So the adaptation to be able to digest lactose into adulthood was advantageous. In other parts of the world where milk didn't make up a large part of the traditional diet, less than 30 percent of the population retains the ability to produce lactase into adulthood.

Superficially, it would seem simple: for those who make lactase, milk and dairy is good, and for those who don't make lactase, milk and dairy aren't so good. But it turns out that lactose isn't always a problem, even for those who don't produce lactase.

Why would that be? Because if you cannot enzymatically digest a carbohydrate it becomes food for the bacteria in your large intestines. In other words, for people who don't produce lactase, lactose is effectively *fiber*. It feeds the bacteria in the large intestine. Not only that, but it preferentially feeds one of the most beneficial classes of bacteria in the human digestive system: *Bifodobacterium* (Parche, et al., 2006).

Those who do not produce the lactase enzyme fall into two categories. One group eats dairy without problem. The other group avoids dairy because it can cause digestive discomfort for them.

What is the difference between these two groups? The answer would seem to be their gut microbiome (i.e. their "beneficial bacteria"), which is something that is modifiable by way of diet.

Those who experience digestive discomfort don't have large numbers of the bifidobacteria that digest lactose (and produce short chain fatty acids that improve the health of the intestines). It's the very same reason many people who are accustomed to eating a low fiber diet will experience digestive problems if they suddenly eat large amounts of fiber.

Remember, for those who don't produce lactase, lactose is effectively fiber. And a cup of milk contains about 12 grams of lactose "fiber". That means that for a person who doesn't produce lactose, a pint of milk contains 24 grams of fiber!

But there's good news. Those who cannot tolerate large amounts of lactose can usually develop tolerance simply by regularly eating lactose (Szilagyi, 2015). The most comfortable way to achieve that is to introduce lactose in small amounts and increase slowly as the number of bifidobacteria in the digestive system increase.

In summary, lactose is a natural sugar that is perfectly healthy for those who can digest it. For those who are unable to produce lactase, large amounts of lactose without digestive support (lactase and/or bacteria that digest lactose) can be problematic. However, fermentation, and aging (cheese) can greatly improve the digestibility of milk, even for those who don't produce lactase. And regular consumption of lactose feeds bifidobacteria that digest lactose, producing health effects and increasing lactose tolerance in most people.

DAIRY CAUSES CANCER

In recent times, the rumor has been spreading that claims that dairy causes cancer. This myth is scary enough that it is causing some people to reconsider dairy. So let's dig in and see if it is actually true. Does dairy actually cause cancer?

First of all, what is the basis of the claim that dairy causes cancer? It turns out that there are perhaps two major sources. For one, there is the claim popularized by Loren Cordain, author of *The Paleo Diet*, which is that a growth factor in milk called betacellulin may cause cancer. Others argue that another growth factor – insulin growth factor 1 (IGF-1) – found in dairy causes cancer. For our purposes, we'll consider these two arguments to be essentially the same – that some growth factor in dairy causes cancer. Secondly, there are some interpretations of data, such as Colin Campbell's *The China Study*, that purport that cancer rates are higher in populations with high rates of dairy consumption. Let's look at each of these and see what the truth may be.

First, let's look at the argument that claims that growth factors in milk cause cancer. Loren Cordain published a newsletter in which he cited 25 studies that he claims provide evidence that dairy causes cancers. I am indebted to Chris Masterjohn for his article, *Does Milk Cause Cancer?* (Masterjohn, 2007), in which he does an excellent job analyzing the claim by looking at the actual studies cited by Cordain. So what do the studies show? Let's take a look.

Both betacellulin and IGF-1 are present in whey and many whey products. The research shows that whey is actually *protective* against cancer. For example, in a paper titled, *Whey proteins in cancer prevention* (Bounous, Batist, & Gold, 1991), the authors state that "epidemiological and experimental studies suggest that dietary milk products may exert an

27

inhibitory effect on the development of several types of tumors". So already there is evidence strongly opposing the theory that dairy causes cancer.

Furthermore, studies have shown that conjugated linoleic acid (CLA), present in dairy fat, exerts a protective effect against some cancers. So even if growth factors such as betacellulin and IGF-1, when taken in isolation, *may* produce cancer growth, it seems that there are other highly protective factors in whole milk that not only prevent the growth factors from producing cancer, but may sometimes help prevent or reverse cancer from other causes.

When it comes to breast, colon, lung, stomach, and pancreatic cancers, the papers cited by Cordain fail to show any evidence of a connection between dairy consumption and cancer. In fact, many actually demonstrate the possibility that dairy consumption, particularly full-fat dairy, provides a protective effect in the case of many types of cancer.

However, there are two types of cancer that do have a positive correlation with low- or non-fat dairy consumption. Both ovarian and prostate cancers occur more frequently in populations who consume low-fat dairy. However, it turns out to be disingenuous to blame dairy, per se. As the authors of one study write, "A high calcium intake, mainly from dairy products, may increase prostate cancer risk by lowering concentrations of 1,25-dihydroxyvitamin $D_3[1,25(OH)_2D_3]$, a hormone thought to protect against prostate cancer." (Chan, et al., 2001) In other words, it's not dairy, it's low vitamin D. And guess what? Full-fat dairy protects against both prostate and ovarian cancer. So the moral of the story is: don't drink large amounts of skim milk and stay indoors all the time. Instead, eat some butter and get some sun. It's good for the ovaries and prostate.

The growth hormone in dairy theory of cancer is bunk.

Next, let's look at the claims made by Campbell and how they stand up to reality. Campbell is famously pro-vegan, and he is a darling among the plant-based diet contingent because he claims in *The China Study* that there is strong evidence that animal protein causes cancer, heart disease, diabetes, and all other forms of ill health. He is particularly anti-casein, and he generalizes his anti-casein stance to dairy and then to all animal proteins. But is he right?

In a word, no, he is not right. Denise Minger, author of *Death by Food Pyramid* has written some extensive critiques of Campbell's conclusions in *The China Study*. And she specifically addresses some of Campbell's claims regarding dairy causing cancer. Campbell has an ax to grind with regard to dairy, but it's not clear that he's got any legs to stand on, so to speak. His argument is two-fold. First, he argues that in his laboratory he was able to "turn on and turn off cancer growth" in rats using casein, a protein from milk. Secondly, he argues that the numbers in *The China Study* demonstrate that dairy consumption positively correlates to cancer in populations. Let's look at these arguments.

The first argument is, perhaps, the more convincing of the two. Granted, lab rats are not humans, but nonetheless, being able to "turn on and turn off cancer growth" using casein is pretty impressive. Campbell is referring to a study he performed (Dunaif & Campbell, 1987). The study actually shows something different than what Campbell claims. It shows that rats made sick with carcinogens who were fed a 20 percent casein diet for a full 12 weeks showed greater preneoplastic lesions (which usually precede tumor growth) than those who were fed less casein. Well, sort of. Actually, the rats that were fed a low-protein diet for the entire duration of the experiment didn't fare much better, it turns out. That is a far cry from casein causing cancer.

The main problem with Campbell's assertion is that it just doesn't hold up in the test of the real world. In the real world, dairy consumption does not seem to contribute to cancer. Sure, industrially processed, isolated casein fed in ridiculous amounts to lab rats for 12 weeks straight may not offer perfect protection against exposure to known carcinogens. But then if that provides proof that casein is carcinogenic, we might as well claim that water is carcinogenic, because I bet that the rats were given water, too.

Finally, Chris Masterjohn offers a critique of Campbell's rat study citations, pointing out that in actuality, casein *is* protective against the effects of aflatoxin (the carcinogen used in the studies). It turns out that in the Indian study that sparked Campbell's interest, the rats exposed to aflatoxin and fed a 5 percent casein diet all died before the conclusion of the study. On the other hand, the rats fed a 20 percent casein diet were still alive. Sure, they had neoplastic lesions, but then again, they were exposed repeatedly to a known carcinogen at insane and completely unnatural levels. And unlike the low-protein diet rats, the high-protein diet rats were still alive at the end.

Campbell makes the weaker claim that the statistical numbers that he used to generate his *China Study* results indicate that animal protein (including dairy) causes cancer. This is a subject that we'll look at in more detail later in the book, but for now, let's just address the dairy issue, specifically. Denise Minger appropriately points out that Campbell neatly omits from his study the only populations in China that actually consume dairy. Of those groups, one stands out in particular because of the large amount of dairy the group consumes. The Tuoli receive more than half of their calories from dairy. And do they have increased cases of cancer? According to the numbers, no, they do not.

In conclusion, there is simply no evidence that dairy causes cancer. In fact, there is considerable evidence that dairy, particularly full-fat dairy, is protective. Vitamin D deficiency, which can be exacerbated by large amounts of calcium in the absence of dairy fat, does correlate positively with ovarian and prostate cancer. So for those who stay indoors and don't supplement with vitamin D, drinking large amounts of non-fat milk is probably a bad idea. But then again, so is eating a lot of broccoli, which is also a bioavailable source of calcium. The negative effects of too much calcium and not enough vitamin D seems to be offset by adequate dairy fat consumption.

DAIRY IS NOT A GOOD SOURCE OF CALCIUM

Many vegan advocates have been pushing the myth that dairy is a poor source of calcium for some time now. The argument usually is that dairy actually leaches more calcium from the bones than it provides. Because it gets repeated often enough and because those who repeat and listen to the argument are willing believers, the myth continues to be spread. But is it true? Let's take a look.

The myth is founded upon the idea that protein causes calcium loss. The first report that suggested this possibility was from 1920 in a paper titled *Calcium Requirement of Maintenance in Man* (Sherman, 1920). The researchers observed that people who eat high protein diets excrete more calcium in their urine when compared to those who eat a low protein diet. Subsequently, dozens of studies have verified this finding. And based on this fact, some people have decided that the calcium being excreted in the urine must be coming from the bones, weakening the bones over time and leading to conditions such as osteoporosis. That is quite a leap, and it turns out that it is unfounded.

Numerous studies show that higher protein intake correlates positively with *increased* bone density (Dawson-Hughes & Harris, 2002). So how could this be? In a paper titled *Low Protein Intake: The Impact on Calcium and Bone Homeostasis in Humans* (Kerstetter, O'Brien, & Insogna, Low Protein Intake: The Impact on Calcium and Bone Homeostasis in Humans, 2003), the authors conclude that higher protein intake leads to increased calcium absorption. Therefore, the additional calcium excreted in the urine likely is due to increased calcium absorption rather than leaching calcium from the bones.

As it turns out, dairy really is one of the very best sources of calcium. Although plant-based diet advocates like to present the idea that plant sources of calcium are superior to dairy, the reality seems to be that they are, in fact, about equivalent in terms of bioavailability. Only about 35 percent of the calcium in most dairy foods is absorbable. But the same is true of the calcium in most plant foods, as well. The calcium in spinach is about 35 percent bioavailable, while a few brassicas like kale come in closer to 50 percent.

But here's the rub. Dairy contains *vastly* more calcium than do vegetables. A single cup of milk contains 300 mg, whereas it would require three quarters of a *pound* of spinach to contain as much. And while kale is more bioavailable, it has far less calcium than does spinach. Theoretically, it is possible to obtain adequate calcium from a plant-based diet, but it requires eating a *lot* of spinach, kale, and other plant sources of calcium. Several pounds every day. And although vegan advocates like to claim otherwise, the evidence as reported in a paper titled *Comparative fracture risk in vegetarians and nonvegetarians in EPIC-Oxford* (Appleby, Roddam, Allen, & Key, 2007) concludes: "The higher fracture risk in the vegans appeared to be a consequence of their considerably lower mean calcium intake. An adequate calcium intake is essential for bone health, irrespective of dietary preferences."

Supplements are a viable option for many people to provide adequate calcium. However, it would appear that in the absence of adequate dietary protein, bone density loss is more likely to occur. By all appearances, full-fat dairy is the best source of calcium, particularly for the purposes of improving bone health, since it contains not only lots of calcium, but also protein and fat-soluble vitamins that contribute to bone health.

DAIRY CAUSES INSULIN RESISTANCE AND DIABETES

These days, many people are looking to find reasons to dislike dairy, and they're digging deep. Both the vegan and the paleo contingents love to find reasons to support their ideological hatred of dairy. And one of the myths that has been stirred up of late is the idea that dairy causes insulin resistance and diabetes.

When I read this myth, it is never accompanied by science that shows that dairy actually causes insulin resistance, or that dairy consumption correlates positively to insulin resistance. But it is often accompanied by a theory that sounds very science-*like* for why the person perpetuating the myth believes that dairy *ought* to cause insulin resistance. And that theory is usually founded upon an incorrect understanding of the causes of insulin resistance. Namely, many people seem to believe that insulin resistance is caused by repeated insulin spikes in the blood. In other words, they believe that eating foods that produce a strong insulin response will eventually lead to insulin resistance – as if the insulin sensitivity simply gets blunted by insulin responses after eating. But it turns out that (as we've already seen earlier in this book) it doesn't seem to work that way.

If insulin resistance was caused by repeated insulin responses, then it would be easy to believe that dairy would cause insulin resistance. That is because dairy produces an unusually large insulin response that is not explained simply by the total levels of sugar and protein it contains (carbohydrates and protein are both known to trigger insulin secretion). Instead, it would seem that the specific *quality* of protein, specifically the amino acid structure of whey protein, causes the insulin response. As a result, milk produces an insulin response similar to that of white bread, despite the fact that the glycemic effects are dramatically lower.

One of the properties of insulin is that it is strongly anabolic. That means that it prevents the breakdown of protein in the body and instead favors growth. Therefore, it makes perfect sense that dairy should produce a strong insulin response, since milk is ideally suited for the needs of rapidly-growing young mammals. Dairy is well-known among athletes and bodybuilders who want to grow muscle mass and strength as being a superior food, in part because of its anabolic effects. So the mere fact that dairy prompts an insulin response is not in and of itself problematic. In fact, it can be very good for health.

Some interesting studies show that the insulin response of dairy may actually be helpful in reducing markers of insulin resistance. For example, in one such paper the authors conclude that whey protein "contributes to blood glucose control by both insulin-dependent and insulin-independent mechanisms." (Akhavan, Luhovyy, Brown, Cho, & Anderson, 2010)

Other studies show that dairy consumption improves glucose control and insulin sensitivity. For example, the Harvard School of Public Health issued a press release in 2010 stating that trans-palmitoleic acid in milk may "substantially reduce the risk of type 2 diabetes." Other studies show an inverse relationship between dairy consumption and insulin resistance, meaning that those who drink a lot of milk have less insulin resistance. There are also studies showing that dairy consumption has no relationship to weight gain (strongly associated with insulin resistance).

In conclusion, while dairy does create a rise in insulin secretion, the evidence is that it lowers the risk of insulin resistance. Those who promote the idea that insulin secretion in response to dairy is a problem for most people misunderstand the role and properties of insulin, as well as the possible causes of insulin resistance. Insulin resistance does not seem to be caused solely by eating foods that create a strong insulin response. Instead, there seem to be other more likely causes, including stress, smoking, lack of sleep, inflammation, and unnaturally high intake of free fructose, to name a few of the possible contributing factors.

DAIRY CAUSES RHEUMATOID ARTHRITIS

Thus far, dietary interventions have shown no consistent ability to improve symptoms in cases of rheumatoid arthritis. Still, the myth that dairy causes rheumatoid arthritis continues to enjoy popularity. Of course, the claim that dairy could cause rheumatoid arthritis is bold and completely out of line with the conventional understanding of what rheumatoid arthritis is. So most likely when people make the claim, what they really mean to suggest is that dairy may be involved in worsening symptoms. So, this is the myth that we'll investigate.

Over the years, a number of studies have looked at the effects of dietary interventions in regard to rheumatoid arthritis. Notably, in a 1983 study (Panush, et al., 1983) a group was placed on a special diet that excluded all additives, preservatives, fruit, red meat, herbs, and dairy. (I can't help but wonder what the heck they ate!) After 10 weeks, the authors reported that "there were no clinically important differences" between the test and control groups.

Other studies have examined the possible role of bovine serum albumin (BSA) present in dairy foods and rheumatoid arthritis. The theory being tested was that humans who develop BSA antibodies may experience rheumatoid arthritis symptoms as a result, since BSA closely resembles human collagen in the joints. What the studies show is that BSA antibodies are common in humans both with and without rheumatoid arthritis, and doesn't seem to be linked to rheumatoid arthritis symptoms.

Although dairy does not seem to cause arthritis flare-ups for most people, there are cases in which removing dairy seems to reduce symptoms. Panush and colleagues reported a case study of one woman who had a worsening of symptoms following dairy consumption. So it is possible that some people with rheumatoid arthritis will benefit from reducing or eliminating dairy, but for the majority of people, there does not seem to be a connection. And in any case, for those who do not have rheumatoid arthritis, there is little reason to believe that dairy could cause the condition.

ANIMAL PROTEIN CAUSES CANCER

In the earlier discussion when we examined the myth that dairy causes cancer, we briefly ran into this myth: that animal protein, in general, causes cancer. This myth was probably initially stoked by Campbell's *The China Study*. Recently, however, the myth received a major shot in the arm when an article in Cell Metabolism (Levine, et al., 2014) reported a positive correlation between high animal protein intake and cancer risk in those between the ages of 50 and 65 (though high animal protein intake was shown to correlate inversely in those 65 and over, meaning it could be protective in that group). So what is going on here? What is the truth?

To begin with, let's look at Campbell's *China Study* claims. He boldly claims that high animal protein intake positively correlates to increased cancer rates. He bases this claim on two things. First, he claims that a series of laboratory tests that he performed on rats demonstrated that high protein intake "switched on" cancer in the rats. Secondly, he claims that his massive epidemiological study shows a positive correlation between populations that eat high protein diets and cancer, whereas those who eat low protein diets have low rates of cancer. Specifically, he singles out *animal* protein as being problematic.

Unfortunately for Campbell, his own rat studies largely disprove his own theory. As Chris Masterjohn points out, in Campbell's own studies in the 1970s, his low-protein (5 percent) rats failed to grow and developed fatty livers. Campbell actually reported in those studies that the low-protein rats developed a massively increased susceptibility to aflatoxin, the carcinogen used to induce cancer. Not only were they more susceptible to aflatoxin, but the toxicity of some pesticides increased by 2100 fold in the low-protein rats! The low-protein rats were suffering from protein deficiency and malnourishment.

The high-protein rats, on the other hand, being fed 20 percent casein, showed a great deal more resilience when compared to the low-protein rats. Campbell exposed the high-protein rats to 5 ppm aflatoxin, but had to use only half the dose with the low-protein rats, because the 5 ppm was lethal to the low-protein group.

Campbell's later studies showed that rats exposed to aflatoxin developed pre-cancerous lesions. There were four groups of rats. Two groups were fed low protein (5 percent) for the first part of the experiment. Two groups were fed high protein (20 percent) for the first part of the experiment. Then, in the second half of the experiment, one group from the low-protein group was switched to a high-protein diet and one group from the high-protein group was switched to a low-protein diet. In other words, there were low-low, low-high, high-low, and high-high groups. What is interesting is that the group that fared the worst *by far* was the low-high group. The low-low group and the high-high groups were fairly similar. And the high-low group fared the best *by far.*

Although it is possible to interpret the data as suggesting that the ideal diet is one that is high in protein in childhood and low in protein in adulthood, it turns out that would be misleading. The reason being that, as we saw in Campbell's earlier studies, extremely low protein (5 percent qualifies as a significant protein deficiency) produces a whole bunch of undesirable effects.

If Campbell's study has any applicability in humans (and that is yet to be seen), it seems extremely unlikely that eating a protein-deficient diet, even if it may offer protection against some types of cancer, is a good idea. And the obvious question remains: if protein intake plays a role in cancer protection, might a moderate protein diet offer the same benefits without producing a protein deficiency? Also, since no one actually eats isolated casein as their sole protein source, might not the effects of a high-casein diet be due to the unnatural and unbalanced exclusive nature of the diet? And might a natural diet containing the balance of amino acids and complementary nutrients found in normal foods offer protection against cancer that a casein diet doesn't?

Furthermore, Campbell makes a point to tell us that a high-casein diet failed to offer protection against aflatoxin, while vegetable proteins tested (namely, gluten) seemed to prevent pre-cancerous lesion formation. But in his own report, he writes that "lysine supplementation of wheat gluten during the postinitiation period enhanced the gamma-glutamyltransferase-positive response to a level comparable with that of the high-quality protein." In other words, adding lysine as found in beans, for example (remember the vegetarian adage to combine beans and rice to get a "complete protein"), produced the same results. By Campbell's own admission, by eating a diet of any sort, so long as the diet supplies sufficient complete protein, the outcomes can be expected to be the same. That is to say that beans and rice will produce the same "carcinogenic" effects as a hamburger.

Campbell's second argument is that the epidemiological study data for *The China Study* showed a strong positive correlation between animal protein intake and diseases of all kinds, including cancers of every sort. But unfortunately for Campbell, the data has now been analyzed by others to show that no such correlation exists. In fact, contrary to Campbell's claim, the data shows a correlation between *vegetable protein* intake and various cancers!

Campbell wasn't strictly fudging the data. Instead, he was using blood cholesterol levels as a proxy for animal protein consumption. And because blood cholesterol levels correlate positively to various diseases, he jumped to the (incorrect) conclusion that animal protein intake was responsible. But it turns out that he was wrong. Blood cholesterol levels can be influenced by a great many factors, and animal protein intake isn't a strong factor. And, in any case, for all we know, high blood cholesterol levels are a consequence of various diseases, or there may be absolutely no connection at all.

Finally, a study published more recently in Cell Metabolism gave rise to a bunch of sensationalistic headlines such as: "Diets high in meat, eggs and dairy could be as harmful to health as smoking." The study looked at data for over 6,000 people over age 50, and attempted to find the relationship between protein intake and disease.

The study began with a hypothesis: researchers found that among people with a particular condition known as growth hormone receptor deficiency, and among those who practice caloric restriction (without malnutrition), there were no cancer mortalities or cases of diabetes. So they speculated that this may be due to reductions in growth factors or the effects of growth factors. They wanted to see if protein restriction might produce the same sorts of effects.

Despite the sensationalistic way in which the study has been handled by media, the authors of the study are reasonably even-handed. The paper even states that "protein restriction **or restriction of particular amino acids, such as methionine and tryptophan**, may explain part of the effects of calorie restriction and GHRD mutations on longevity and disease risk." In other words, the effects of protein restriction may be obtainable simply by reducing (or offsetting) particular amino acids.

What is of note is that several studies have now shown that restriction of methionine alone can produce many of the same benefits of caloric restriction in terms of longevity and protection from disease. But perhaps even more importantly, a 2011 study shows that (at least in rats) simply supplementing a diet with the amino acid glycine offers all the same benefits, even without having to restrict methionine (Brind, et al., 2011).

Methionine is found in large amounts in muscle meats in particular, but approximately 50 percent of the protein in an animal is collagen (gelatin), which is very high in glycine. The implication here is that eating the whole animal or simply supplementing with gelatin may offer major health benefits and protect against cancer.

Finally, the study only looked at adults age 50 and older. The results suggested that eating large amounts of methionine-rich protein correlates to increased cancer risk for those between 50 and 65, but it correlates to *decreased* cancer risk in those over 65. So a large segment of the population studied may potentially benefit from eating lots of methionine-rich protein, and we have no idea what correlations may exist in younger populations.

In conclusion, the idea that animal protein causes cancer is extremely weak. It seems likely in many cases that moderate or high protein may be protective against cancer. And in any cases where it is not, protective effects may be had by either reducing methionine-rich protein sources or supplementing with glycine-rich proteins.

PROTEIN CAUSES OSTEOPOROSIS

One of the protein (often cast specifically as anti-animal protein) myths in circulation is the myth that (sufficient) dietary protein causes osteoporosis. However, as we'll see, it turns out that quite the opposite may be true. So the typical suggestion that people should reduce (animal) protein intake in order to reduce osteoporosis risk may be extremely harmful. Let's look at the evidence.

You may recall from an earlier section that some researchers have noticed short-term increases in calcium excretion in the urine of people who eat high protein diets. This observation has led many to (incorrectly) assume that some mechanism of a high-protein diet must cause calcium to be pulled from the bones, leading to osteoporosis. But you may also recall that it has been shown that a more likely explanation is that high-protein diets tend to increase calcium absorption, leading to an increase in total calcium. It may then be that the increased calcium excretion is explained simply by the increased absorption.

In any case, regardless of the exact reasons for the differences in calcium in the urine, the studies repeatedly show that sufficient and even "high" protein diets not only do not correlate positively to osteoporosis, but they actually correlate to *improved* bone density.

A review published in the American Journal of Clinical Nutrition stated that "intakes of both calcium and protein must be adequate to fully realize the benefit of each nutrient on bone. Optimal protein intake for bone health is likely higher than current recommended intakes, particularly in the elderly. Concerns about dietary protein increasing urinary calcium appear to be offset by increases in absorption. Likewise, concerns about the impact of protein on acid production appear to be minor compared with the alkalinizing effects of fruits and vegetables." (Heaneyy & Layman, 2008)

Another review published in 2011 came to a similar conclusion, stating that "dietary protein works synergistically with calcium to improve calcium retention and bone metabolism. The recommendation to intentionally restrict dietary protein to improve bone health is unwarranted, and potentially even dangerous to those individuals who consume inadequate protein." (Kerstetter, Kenny, & Insogna, Dietary protein and skeletal health: a review of recent human research., 2011)

Many studies have demonstrated that, particularly in the elderly, low protein intake correlates with loss in bone density and increased risk for fractures. They also show that many elderly people are not eating enough protein.

The connection between restrictive eating disorders and bone loss has long been known by those who study eating disorders. Malnutrition, but perhaps *particularly* insufficient protein coupled with insufficient minerals, seems to contribute to bone loss.

The myth that protein causes osteoporosis is just that, a myth, and a dangerous one at that. Sufficient quality protein intake seems to be essential for bone health. Of course, sufficient protein is not the only factor. Also important are calcium, vitamin D, vitamin K, trace minerals, muscle mass, and adequate movement, among other things.

FOOD COMBINING

The food combining myth has been circulating in various forms for a long time. I'm not sure where or when it originated. Food combining was advocated by William Hay in the 1920s with the Hay Diet. And Herbert Shelton promoted the ideas in the 1930s. Food combining got a major shot in the arm with the publication of Fit for Life in the 1980s, a New York Times best seller. More recently, there's the Body Ecology Diet program, which is popular and advocates for food combining. Even the likes of Dr. Mercola have advocated for the idea.

The premise of food combining is that different types of foods digest differently and that combining them "incorrectly" will wreak havoc on the digestive system, leading to all kinds of health problems from heartburn to cancer. There are a variety of food combining rules, but the most common are as follows:

• Never combine fruit with any non-fruits, but most fruit can be combined with other fruits
   • Never combine melon with anything else
   • Never combine dairy with anything else
   • Never combine protein with starch
   • Never combine sugar (as in fruit) with starch

There are plenty of other variations, including rules about how to combine acid fruits with non-acid fruits and so forth. But the preceding rules capture the essence of most food combining systems.

The reasons given for *why* food combining matters vary, but they are always fairly similar, and the most elegant explanation concerns two matters. First, it is claimed that different types of foods digest in different pH environments – protein in an acidic environment and carbohydrates in an alkaline environment. Therefore, it is suggested that for this reason, protein and carbohydrates should be eaten separately. Secondly, it is claimed that different foods have different transit times when eaten alone and therefore should not be combined, because eating them together will cause one or the other to rot or ferment. Let's look at these arguments.

First, it is true that protein and carbohydrates require different pH environments in order to digest. But the argument that they should therefore be eaten separately actually falls flat on its face. Here's why. Protein begins to be digested in the stomach, which is a highly acidic environment. Eating protein actually causes a further acidification of the stomach to anywhere between a pH of 1 and 3. The low pH is necessary for the protease enzyme pepsin to be active. Pepsin mixes with the protein and breaks it apart into tiny, tiny pieces. It breaks the proteins into smaller proteins. Once that process is complete, the stomach empties into the small intestines.

As the stomach contents (which are acidic) empty into the small intestines, the body secretes bicarbonate, which neutralizes and slightly alkalinizes the chyme from the stomach. This is essential because the small intestines must be alkaline in order for the pancreatic enzymes to function. The pancreatic enzymes include enzymes for digesting fat, protein, and carbohydrates. The enzymes work on the chyme to break it down into sugars, amino acids, and fatty acids that the body can absorb. And, interestingly, the more acidic the stomach contents, the more enzymes the pancreas will secrete, including enzymes to digest carbohydrates.

So it turns out that no matter what we eat, the pH of the stomach is low (acid) and the pH of the small intestines is slightly alkaline. This is true whether one eats fruit alone or meat alone or combines everything together. And because eating protein can prompt greater enzyme secretion in the small intestines (indirectly by lowering the pH of the stomach), it turns out that eating protein and carbohydrates together probably increases the absorption of carbohydrates. So this is a big fail for food combining, thus far.

But what about the argument that combining foods may cause some to rot or ferment? Well, sorry, Dr. Mercola, but it's not true. The extremely acidic environment of the stomach completely prevents fermentation. Anyone who has ever canned food knows that an acidic medium prevents spoilage. Think about pickled cucumbers in vinegar, for example. The pH of the stomach is even lower than the pH required to prevent spoilage of canned food. So the potatoes you eat with steak aren't going to rot in the stomach in the few hours they are in there.

Once the chyme enters the small intestines, the pancreatic enzymes begin to break everything down. Nothing is going to ferment for a few reasons. For one, the enzymes are breaking everything down and it is getting absorbed. For another thing, there's nothing to ferment the sugars, since there should be no bacteria in the small intestines, and because anaerobic fermentation doesn't happen in the intestines. So once again, big fail for food combining.

In conclusion, food combining simply doesn't have any real merit. Humans have evolved over a very long time eating different foods together in the same meal, and our digestive systems are well adapted to it. In fact, there is good evidence that eating different foods together at the same time is actually *better* than eating them apart from one another. Of course, some people may have problems with low stomach acid, for example, which can result in some digestive problems. In those cases, eating a low protein diet may seem to alleviate some of the symptoms. But in the long run, it would be best to increase stomach acid production to healthy levels rather than avoiding protein. In fact, eating more protein may be one way to improve stomach acid production. And protein tastes better with carbohydrates. Dessert is good after dinner. And all of it together improves digestive function.

MEAT ROTS IN THE COLON

One of the myths that gets propagated, particularly by vegan advocates, is the idea that meat rots in the colon. This image is designed to be unappetizing in order to put one off of eating meat. But the reality is that it simply isn't true.

We'll keep this short and sweet since it doesn't require much to thoroughly debunk the myth that meat rots in the colon. As we've seen in the previous section, protein digestion begins in the stomach. Once you eat protein, the stomach pH drops dramatically to somewhere in the 1 to 3 range. The pH has to be less than 3 in order to activate pepsin, which is the protein-digesting enzyme that works in the stomach.

Pepsin is a powerful enzyme. In several hours, it can thoroughly break down just about any protein you throw at it, including sizeable chunks of protein swallowed whole. Pepsin breaks apart proteins into smaller proteins until all the protein is in little, tiny bits, forming a liquid called chyme.

At that point, the stomach empties into the small intestines, where it is buffered by bicarbonate. The bicarbonate raises the pH to be slightly alkaline so that the pancreatic enzymes can work. Among the pancreatic enzymes that the body secretes are proteases that further break down the remaining proteins in the chyme. The proteins get broken into amino acids, which are then absorbed through the small intestines.

The result? By the time the chyme reaches the colon, the protein has been almost entirely absorbed. No meat remains.

To be fair, there are some people who have difficulty digesting some types of protein. For example, as we've seen earlier in the book, some people do have difficulty digesting some components of casein, which is one type of protein from milk. But perhaps the protein that causes the most problems for most people happens to be a *plant* protein – gliadin – from wheat. Ironically, meat proteins are among the easiest to digest. So while some proteins may make it to the colon, meat proteins are the least likely to travel that far.

Does meat rot in the colon? Nope. But fiber does. Though you don't hear a lot of people warning about the dangers of rotting fiber (because it's beneficial).

SATURATED FAT CAUSES CARDIOVASCULAR DISEASE

The most common myth about saturated fat is that it causes cardiovascular disease. This myth is *still* pushed by organizations such as the American Heart Association. But is it true? Let's take a look.

The theory that saturated fat may cause cardiovascular disease was popularized by a man named Ancel Keys. Despite the fact that many people who have seen through the saturated fat myth now like to demonize Keys, it turns out that Keys wasn't such a bad guy. He made many important contributions to our knowledge of human nutrition, and it turns out that his hypothesis was actually founded on good data. The data he collected really did demonstrate a positive correlation between saturated fat intake and cardiovascular disease.

The trouble with the conclusion Keys drew is multifaceted. Denise Minger has written a lovely article in which she pulls apart the problems with the conclusion, relying heavily on a critique written in 1957 by two men named Yerushalmy and Hilleboe (Yerushalmy & Hillboe, 1957). They point out that while countries with higher levels of saturated fat available have higher rates of reported cardiovascular disease, overall they have considerably lower rates of disease when compared to countries with lower levels of saturated fat available. They also point out that higher levels of saturated fat correlate with wealth in the data. And they go on to suggest that less wealthy countries were likely grossly under-reporting cardiovascular disease deaths, instead classifying them as something else.

The real wrench in the works, however, is that the data Keys was working from was simply a report of what food existed in a country. He wasn't looking at what people *actually* were eating. So at the end of the day, although Keys' graphs may be interesting, they didn't tell us anything about real world trends.

Subsequent to Keys' publication, he landed a position on the board of the American Heart Association, and only then did the recommendation to limit dietary saturated fat intake start making its way into mainstream channels. Since then, there's been a steady stream of propaganda warning us to eat less saturated fat. But is this suggestion backed up by good science?

Nope. It's not. And now the evidence is mounting that saturated fat is not a problem. In 2010, a massive meta-analysis project looked at nearly 350,000 subjects and concluded that "there is no significant evidence for concluding that dietary saturated fat is associated with an increased risk of CHD [stroke] or CVD [cardiovascular disease]." (Siri-Tarino, Sun, Hu, & Krauss, 2010)

A former president of the American College of Cardiology and former advocate of the saturated fat myth is now quoted as saying, "The low-fat, high-carbohydrate diet may well have played an unintended role in the current epidemics of obesity, lipid abnormalities, type 2 diabetes, and metabolic syndromes. This diet can no longer be defended by appeal to the authority of prestigious medical organizations." (Weinberg, 2004)

And a recent publication in *Annals of Internal Medicine* performed a meta-analysis of an even larger group of people and concluded that "current evidence does not clearly support cardiovascular guidelines that encourage high consumption of polyunsaturated fatty acids and low consumption of total saturated fats." (Chowdhury, et al., 2014)

Chris Masterjohn put together an excellent analysis of the only high-quality human studies that have been done looking at saturated fat and cardiovascular disease, and he showed that those studies demonstrated absolutely no link at all. In fact, in the L.A. Veteran's Trial, the evidence was that the saturated fat group had *fewer* overall deaths (from all causes) despite the fact that the saturated fat group had more heavy smokers (a known health risk) and that the study design accidentally made the saturated fat group deficient in vitamin E (also a known risk). So all things considered, it would even be reasonable to consider the possibility that saturated fat could be *protective*.

Despite the diehards who are clinging to a sinking ship, the saturated fat causes cardiovascular disease myth has lost credibility. There does not appear to be any cardiovascular risk associated with *natural* saturated fat intake from real foods. And, some saturated fat sources such as butter contain important fat-soluble nutrients as well as other factors (like conjugated linoleic acid) that are shown to be protective against a variety of conditions, including cancer.

CHOLESTEROL CAUSES CARDIOVASCULAR DISEASE

Right alongside the saturated fat myth is the cholesterol myth that suggests that dietary cholesterol causes cardiovascular disease. As a result, many people forgo eggs, liver, and other high-cholesterol foods, thinking they are doing the "heart healthy" thing. But is it true?

To begin with, there are two aspects to the theory. First, there is the idea that dietary cholesterol increases blood cholesterol, which is of primary concern to us in this discussion. But then there is the second matter, which is the idea that blood cholesterol levels determine risk for cardiovascular disease. While we're at it, we might as well debunk them both.

To begin with, the notion that dietary cholesterol increases blood cholesterol has absolutely no basis in reality. In fact, even Ancel Keys, the "grandfather of the diet-heart theory," said in 1997 that "there's no connection whatsoever between the cholesterol in food and cholesterol in the blood. And we've known that all along." (Bowden & Sinatra, 2012) So despite the fact that we've been told to avoid eggs, it turns out that eating eggs, liver, or other high-cholesterol foods has essentially no impact on blood cholesterol levels.

The theory of dietary cholesterol causing atherosclerosis originated, perhaps, from some *rabbit* studies in which the researchers fed (oxidized) cholesterol to rabbits and demonstrated increases in health problems in the rabbits. Consider for a moment that rabbits are naturally herbivores. Adding cholesterol to an herbivore's diet is likely to produce health problems. Add substantial oxidized cholesterol to *anyone's* diet and it's probably going to cause problems. But does this translate to humans eating actual food? No, it does not.

The Framingham Heart Study demonstrated that dietary cholesterol has no impact on rates of cardiovascular disease. Furthermore, the overwhelming evidence of the studies measuring the effects of lowering blood cholesterol levels indicates that it is not an effective way to reduce cardiovascular disease.

In fact, there is considerable evidence that lowering blood cholesterol levels leads to increased risk of a variety of diseases. This has been concluded by a number of studies, including the Framingham Heart Study, the Honolulu Heart Program, and the Japanese Lipid Intervention Trial. (Thanks to Chris Kresser for bringing these studies to attention.)

In conclusion, there is no evidence that dietary cholesterol leads to cardiovascular disease. And there is even evidence that lowering blood cholesterol (through drugs or other means) is a bad idea that not only doesn't improve cardiovascular health, but actually worsens health overall. Then again, if you're a rabbit, you may want to lay off the pure oxidized cholesterol.

SATURATED FAT CAUSES INSULIN RESISTANCE

Almost as what appears to be a last ditch effort to demonize saturated fat, many are now spreading the myth that saturated fat causes insulin resistance. But is it true?

This matter seems a bit complicated. From what I can find, the studies that are often cited as "proof" that saturated fat causes insulin resistance merely show that unnatural applications of saturated free fatty acids to rat livers can produce insulin resistance in the rat livers. While this is interesting (and horrific for the rats), it certainly doesn't prove anything about the effects of natural dietary saturated fats in humans. So let's look at what the studies have to say about the effects of saturated fats in human trials.

Thanks to Stephan Guyenet, I found a paper that states that until the year 2008, only one study in 15 had shown any correlation between saturated fat intake and insulin resistance. That one study, the KANWU study, ran for three months and included 162 participants. One group was fed mostly saturated fats and the other group mostly monounsaturated fats. And despite the conclusion reached by the authors ("decreasing saturated fatty acid and increasing monounsaturated fatty acid improves insulin sensitivity"), the actual reported results were statistically insignificant. There was essentially no difference between the two groups.

Another study compared two groups (20 subjects total), one eating mostly saturated fat and the other eating mostly monounsaturated fat (along with other foods). The study concluded that there were no differences in insulin sensitivity between the two groups. (Dijk, et al., 2009)

In a 2011 study that included 417 subjects – the LIPGENE study – the authors concluded that saturated fat had no negative impact on insulin sensitivity. They also concluded that supplementation with omega-3 fatty acids improved some markers. (Tierney, et al., 2011)

In conclusion, there simply is no evidence that saturated fat contributes to insulin resistance.

SATURATED FAT CAUSES INFLAMMATION

Still beating a poor, dead horse, the anti-saturated fat camp desperately wants to find something – *anything* – bad to pin on saturated fat. And so now the latest myth is that saturated fat causes inflammation. Since inflammation is now linked intimately with just about every type of disease from diabetes to heart disease, the implication here is that saturated fat is very, very bad. But is it true?

It turns out that, like so many things, what has happened is that some media outlets and some people with an ideological standpoint to prop up have latched on to some very preliminary rat study results and decided that the studies prove something that they do not. The studies in question have simply shown that saturated fatty acids in rat brains may play a role in inflammatory cytokine cascades, and that monounsaturated fatty acids seem to be protective. To leap from that to the conclusion that dietary saturated fats found in natural foods will cause major inflammatory responses in humans is just too big of a chasm to bridge.

As we've already seen, saturated fat is not linked to conditions such as insulin resistance or cardiovascular disease. In fact, there is even some evidence that saturated fat may be protective in some cases. And these conditions are closely linked with inflammation. In fact, the link is so close that many now suspect that inflammation may be the primary driver of the conditions. So if saturated fat produces inflammation in humans, we would expect to see that saturated fat intake would be positively correlated with these conditions, which it is not. So in the real world, the saturated fat causes inflammation theory seems to fall flat on its face.

Just as importantly, it seems worth remembering that, in the real world, there is no such thing as pure saturated fat. In laboratory settings, researchers have produced fully-saturated coconut oil and used that to produce essential fatty acid deficiencies. But real, natural coconut oil can't produce essential fatty acid deficiencies. Why? Because it contains a natural complement of fatty acids, including both saturated and unsaturated fatty acids.

In the real world, highly saturated fats such as coconut oil or butter contain not only saturated fats but also unsaturated fats and other substances that offer health benefits. For example, butter contains butyric acid, which has been shown in both animal and human studies to possess an impressive array of anti-inflammatory properties. Butter and many animal fats such as beef tallow contain conjugated linoleic acid, an unsaturated fatty acid that has anti-inflammatory and immune-boosting properties. And even though fats like butter and tallow contain a lot of saturated fat, they also contain a lot of *mono*unsaturated fat, which the studies repeatedly show is anti-inflammatory.

In conclusion, there is no good evidence that eating saturated fat causes inflammation in humans. And, it turns out that many natural sources of saturated fat contain anti-inflammatory properties. There seems to be little cause for concern. You can probably eat butter with impunity.

SALT CAUSES HIGH BLOOD PRESSURE

The myth that salt increases blood pressure has been around for a while – likely at least as far back as 1904 when some doctors in France found that six subjects who had high blood pressure also happened to eat a lot of salt. Then in the 1940s, a researcher named Kemper was able to show that reducing salt intake in some people led to drops in blood pressure. Studies continued and in the 1970s, a man named Dahl fed rats what would amount to more than a pound of salt for an adult human and cited that as proof that salt causes high blood pressure.

As a result of the myth that salt causes high blood pressure, many people have been advised to limit their salt intake. Ironically, many people who have high blood pressure actually crave salt. Nonetheless, many obey the orders and restrict salt. The question is, is there a payoff? Does salt substantially increase blood pressure? And if so, is that associated with any increase in diseases?

The conclusions from the rather extensive studies that have been conducted in this matter are categorical. In no way does salt restriction offer any benefits to blood pressure or offer protection from disease. In fact, some studies conclude that increased salt intake correlates to decreased risk of various diseases, including heart disease!

The Cochrane Collaborative, a non-for-profit research organization, published two reviews of trials – one in 2004 and one in 2011 – both of which concluded that there is no benefit in reducing salt intake. In 2011, Cochrane wrote that "cutting down on the amount of salt has no clear benefits in terms of likelihood of dying or experiencing cardiovascular disease."

The Journal of the American Medical Association published a paper in 2011 concluding that "systolic blood pressure, but not diastolic pressure, changes over time aligned with change in sodium excretion, but this association did NOT translate into a higher risk of hypertension or cardiovascular disease complications." (Katarzyna Stolarz-Skrzypek, et al., 2011)

These reports are not alone. There are more than 10 such reports that I have found that draw the same conclusions: increased sodium intake does not cause high blood pressure or higher rates of disease. In fact, some of the studies conclude that reducing sodium intake is correlated to *higher* rates of health problems in some populations.

The body maintains a balance between sodium and potassium. Too little sodium leads to a condition known as hyponatremia. This condition can be brought about in a variety of ways, the most common of which is excessive water intake following prolonged physical exertion, and in some rare cases it can even prove fatal. Unfortunately, a lot of people may be producing mild hyponatremia by greatly reducing or eliminating salt intake coupled with increasing potassium intake (through ingesting more things like green smoothies).

Both sodium and potassium are essential nutrients for human health. Too little of either can cause serious problems. Many people eat too little potassium, creating an imbalance in the sodium to potassium ratio. The ratio can be corrected by limiting sodium intake, of course. But doing so results in deficiencies of *both* nutrients rather than correcting the existing potassium deficiency.

Different people respond differently to salt. Some people are more sensitive to salt than others. But by and large, the evidence suggests that modest salt intake (up to 6 grams of sodium per day) does not cause high blood pressure or diseases.

HAVE NO FEAR

Now that we've taken apart all these myths, what do you do? If you're like a lot of us, you've used these myths to keep yourself under tight dietary control. They provided structure so that you clearly knew which foods were "good" and which were "bad." But without the rules, how will you know how to eat?

Hopefully, you can start to take the fear out of food. Of course, we're all different. What is right for one is not always right for everyone else. But then again, what is right in one moment isn't always right, even for the same person. I mean, sometimes eating chocolate cake is the right thing, but if you tried to eat chocolate cake all the time, you'd probably feel sick.

The thing about the rules and having good foods and bad foods is that it artificially limits the possibilities for meeting your nutritional needs. And in some cases, it restricts so greatly that you cannot meet your nutritional needs. This is particularly true when we eliminate entire categories of food from our diets such as eliminating all sugar (including honey and fruit) or starch, or eliminating all meat or dairy.

By removing the rules, you instead have the radical possibility available to you of eating what your body wants. When you're not overanalyzing everything, it gets easier to simply eat what you want. Of course, we may have all kinds of fears about the implications of eating what we want, but by and large, those fears are unfounded when we actually eat unrestrictedly of real foods.

Many of the so-called experts are now catching on that the rules have tended to make things worse for us in terms of health. The low-fat rules led to increased intake of trans fats and free fructose. The low-sugar rules led people to increased intake of artificial sweeteners. The no-dairy and no-meat rules led people to increased intake of unfermented soy, artificial ingredients, and other unhealthy things. And the low-salt rules led people to eat less salt, which actually is a health risk!

So it turns out that removing the rules is unlikely to have nearly the negative impact that the rules have had. And it also turns out that a lot of the stuff that tastes good is actually pretty good for you. Fruit, honey, butter, cheese, potatoes, salt, red meat, and even sucrose (i.e. sugar) when eaten according to desire are likely to offer health benefits. Who knew?

Stop fearing the food. Eat good food that you actually enjoy eating. And enjoy eating it. Smile. Relax. Sleep enough. Enjoy the outdoors. It's all good for   you.

GET ANOTHER OF MY BOOKS FOR FREE

If you've enjoyed this book, there's more where this one came from. And I'd be delighted to give you another one of my books for free.

My book *Cleansed* is a reader favorite. Here are some of the things reviewers have to say about it:

"[G]et the book and enjoy Joey's gift of explaining and educating through the written word"

"Finally, some sense"

"This book was worth every minute I spent reading it."

"I am so thankful to have found and read this book"

Download your free digital copy of *Cleansed* today by visiting http://joeylotthealth.com/cleansed-free-offer

PLEASE WRITE A REVIEW OF THIS BOOK

If you liked this book, it would be fabulous if you would write a review of it on site of the retailer from which you got the book

I know, I know. You think it doesn't matter. And it is sort of obnoxious that I ask you to take a minute from your valuable time to do something like write a review of this book.

But actually, reviews are really, really helpful. And that's the reason I ask.

See, the way the retailers work is they help potential readers to discover new books, *but only if those books have* recent *reviews*.

So if you liked this book and would like others to be able to discover it, please do take a moment right now to write a review and post it on the site of the retailer from which you got this book. It really does make a difference.

Thank   you.

REFERENCES

Akhavan, T., Luhovyy, B., Brown, P., Cho, C., & Anderson, G. (2010). Effect of premeal consumption of whey protein and its hydrolysate on food intake and postmeal glycemia and insulin responses in young adults. *Am J Clin Nutr*, 966-975.

Allen, B. G., Bhatia, S. K., Anderson, C. M., Eichenberger-Gilmore, J. M., Sibenaller, Z. A., Mapuskar, K. A., . . . Fath, M. A. (2014). Ketogenic diets as an adjuvant cancer therapy: History and potential mechanism. *Redox Biol*, 963-970.

Anderson, G. (1995). Sugars, sweetness, and food intake. *Am J Clin Nutr*, 195S-201S.

Appleby, P., Roddam, A., Allen, N., & Key, T. (2007). Comparative fracture risk in vegetarians and nonvegetarians in EPIC-Oxford. *Eur J Clin Nutr.*, 1400-1406.

Barclay, A. (2008). Glycemic index, glycemic load, and chronic disease risk. *Am J Clin Nutr*, 627-637.

Beck-Nielsen, H., Pedersen, O., & Lindskov, H. (1980). Impaired cellular insulin binding and insulin sensitivity induced by high-fructose feeding in normal subjects. *Am J Clin Nutr*, 273-280.

Bell, S., Grochoski, G., & Clarke, A. (2006). Health implications of milk containing beta-casein with the A2 genetic variant. *Crit Rev Food Sci Nutr*, 93-100.

Black, R., Spence, M., McMahon, R., Cuskelly, G., Ennis, C., McCance, D., . . . Hunter, S. (2006). Effect of eucaloric high- and low-sucrose diets with identical macronutrient profile on insulin resistance and vascular risk: a randomized controlled trial. *Diabetes*, 3566-3572.

Bounous, G., Batist, G., & Gold, P. (1991). Whey proteins in cancer prevention. *Cancer Lett*, 91-94.

Bowden, J., & Sinatra, S. (2012). *The Great Cholesterol Myth*. Fair Winds Press.

Brind, J., Malloy, V., Augie, I., Caliendo, N., Vogelman, J. H., Zimmerman, J. A., & Orentreich, N. (2011). Dietary glycine supplementation mimics lifespan extension by dietary methionine restriction in Fisher 344 rats. *The FASEB Journal*, Supplement 528.2.

Chan, J. M., Stampfer, M. J., Ma, J., Gann, P. H., Gaziano, J. M., & Giovannucci, E. L. (2001). Dairy products, calcium, and prostate cancer risk in the Physicians' Health Study. *Am J Clin Nutr*, 549-554.

Chowdhury, Warnakula, Kunutsor, Crowe, Ward, Johnson, . . . Thompson SG, K. K. (2014). Association of dietary, circulating, and supplement fatty acids with coronary risk: a systematic review and meta-analysis. *Ann Intern Med*, 398-406.

Daher, R., Yazbeck, T., Jaoude, J. B., & Abboud, B. (2009). Consequences of dysthyroidism on the digestive tract and viscera. *World J Gastroenterol*, 2834–2838.

Dawson-Hughes, B., & Harris, S. (2002). Calcium intake influences the association of protein intake with rates of bone loss in elderly men and women. *Am J Clin Nutr*, 773-779.

Dijk, v., Feskens, Bos, Hoelen, Heijligenberg, Bromhaar, . . . Afman. (2009). A saturated fatty acid-rich diet induces an obesity-linked proinflammatory gene expression profile in adipose tissue of subjects at risk of metabolic syndrome. *Am J Clin Nutr*, 1656-1664.

Dunaif, G., & Campbell, T. (1987). Relative contribution of dietary protein level and aflatoxin B1 dose in generation of presumptive preneoplastic foci in rat liver. *J Natl Cancer Inst*, 365-369.

Heaneyy, R. P., & Layman, D. K. (2008). Amount and type of protein influences bone health. *Am J Clin Nutr*, 1567S-1570S .

Katarzyna Stolarz-Skrzypek, M. P., Tatiana Kuznetsova, M. P., Lutgarde Thijs, M., Valérie Tikhonoff, M. P., Jitka Seidlerová, M. P., Tom Richart, M., . . . Edoardo Casiglia, M. P. (2011). Fatal and Nonfatal Outcomes, Incidence of Hypertension, and Blood Pressure Changes in Relation to Urinary Sodium Excretion. *JAMA*, 1777-1785.

Kerstetter, J., Kenny, A., & Insogna, K. (2011). Dietary protein and skeletal health: a review of recent human research. *Curr Opin Lipidol*, 16-20.

Kerstetter, J., O'Brien, K., & Insogna, K. (2003). Low Protein Intake: The Impact on Calcium and Bone Homeostasis in Humans. *J Nutr*, 855S-861S.

King, J. C., & Slavin, J. L. (2013). White Potatoes, Human Health, and Dietary Guidance. *Adv Nutr*, 393S–401S.

Le, A., Lane, A. N., Hamaker, M., Bose, S., Gouw, A., Barbi, J., . . . Lorkiewicz, P. K. (2013). Glucose-independent glutamine metabolism via TCA cycling for proliferation and survival in B-cells. *Cell Metab*, 110-121.

Lê, K., Faeh, D., Stettler, R., Ith, M., Kreis, R., Vermathen, P., . . . Tappy, L. (2006). A 4-wk high-fructose diet alters lipid metabolism without affecting insulin sensitivity or ectopic lipids in healthy humans. *Am J Clin Nutr*, 1374-1379.

Levine, M. E., Suarez, J. A., Brandhorst, S., Balasubramanian, P., Cheng, C.-W., Madia, F., . . . Mirisola, M. G. (2014). Low Protein Intake Is Associated with a Major Reduction in IGF-1, Cancer, and Overall

Mortality in the 65 and Younger but Not Older Population. *Cell Metabolism*, 407-417.

Liljeberg, H., & Björck, I. (1998). Delayed gastric emptying rate may explain improved glycaemia in healthy subjects to a starchy meal with added vinegar. *Eur J Clin Nutr.*, 368-371.

Lindeberg, S., Eliasson, M., Lindahl, B., & Ahrén, B. (1999). Low serum insulin in traditional Pacific Islanders--the Kitava Study. *Metabolism*, 1216-1219.

Lindeberg, S., Nilsson-Ehle, P., Terént, A., Vessby, B., & Scherstén, B. (1994). Cardiovascular risk factors in a Melanesian population apparently free from stroke and ischaemic heart disease: the Kitava study. *J Intern Med*, 331-340.

Maersk, M., Belza, A., Stødkilde-Jørgensen, H., Ringgaard, S., Chabanova, E., Thomsen, H., . . . Richelsen, B. (2012). Sucrose-sweetened beverages increase fat storage in the liver, muscle, and visceral fat depot: a 6-mo randomized intervention study. *Am J Clin Nutr*, 283-289.

Masterjohn, C. (2007, April 30). *Does Milk Cause Cancer? Evaluating the Betacellulin Hypothesis*. Retrieved from Real Milk: http://www.realmilk.com/health/does-milk-cause-cancer/

Meyer, B., van der Merwe, M., Du Plessis, D., de Bruin, E., & Meyer, A. (1971). Some physiological effects of a mainly fruit diet in man. *S Afr Med J*, 191-195.

Moynihan, T. (n.d.). *Cancer Causes*. Retrieved from Mayo Clinic: http://www.mayoclinic.org/diseases-conditions/cancer/in-depth/cancer-causes/art-20044714

Panush, R., Carter, R., Katz, P., Kowsari, B., Longley, S., & Finnie, S. (1983). Diet therapy for rheumatoid arthritis. *Arthritis Rheum*, 462-471.

Parche, S., Beleut, M., Rezzonico, E., Jacobs, D., Arigoni, F., Titgemeyer, F., & Jankovic, I. (2006). Lactose-over-Glucose Preference in

Bifidobacterium longum NCC2705: glcP, Encoding a Glucose Transporter, Is Subject to Lactose Repression. *J Bacteriol*, 1260–1265.

Sargrad, K., Homko, C., Mozzoli, M., & Boden, G. (2005). Effect of high protein vs high carbohydrate intake on insulin sensitivity, body weight, hemoglobin A1c, and blood pressure in patients with type 2 diabetes mellitus. *J Am Diet Assoc*, 573-580.

Schmidt, M., Pfetzer, N., Schwab, M., Strauss, I., & Kämmerer, U. (2011). Effects of a ketogenic diet on the quality of life in 16 patients with advanced cancer: A pilot trial. *Nutr Metab*, 54.

Sherman, H. (1920). Calcium Requirement of Maintenance in Man. *Journal of Biological Chemistry*, 21-27.

Siri-Tarino, P., Sun, Q., Hu, F., & Krauss, R. (2010). Meta-analysis of prospective cohort studies evaluating the association of saturated fat with cardiovascular disease. *Am J Clin Nutr*, 535-546.

Szilagyi, A. (2015). Adaptation to Lactose in Lactase Non Persistent People: Effects on Intolerance and the Relationship between Dairy Food Consumption and Evalution of Diseases. *Nutrients*, 6751-6779.

Tailford, K., Berry, C., Thomas, A., & Campbell, J. (2003). A casein variant in cow's milk is atherogenic. *Atherosclerosis*, 13-19.

Tierney, McMonagle, Shaw, Gulseth, Helal, Saris, . . . Defoort C, W. C.-K.-M. (2011). Effects of dietary fat modification on insulin sensitivity and on other risk factors of the metabolic syndrome--LIPGENE: a European randomized dietary intervention study. *Int J Obes (Lond)*, 800-809.

Weinberg, S. (2004). The diet-heart hypothesis: a critique. *J Am Coll Cardiol.*, 731-733.

Yago, M., Frymoyer, A., Smelick, G., Frassetto, L., Budha, N., Dresser, M., . . . Benet, L. (2013). Gastric Re-acidification with Betaine HCl in Healthy Volunteers with Rabeprazole-Induced Hypochlorhydria. *Mol Pharm*, 4032-4037.

Yerushalmy, J., & Hillboe, H. (1957). Fat in the diet and mortality from heart disease; a methodologic note. *N Y State J Med*, 2343-2354.

Zhang, W., Miao, J., Wang, S., & Zhang, Y. (2013). The protective effects of beta-casomorphin-7 against glucose -induced renal oxidative stress in vivo and vitro. *PLoS One*, e63472.

ABOUT THE AUTHOR

Joey Lott lives in New Mexico on a small homestead with his family. His website can be found at www.joeylotthealth.com.

Made in the USA
Lexington, KY
15 August 2016